Conquering Your Insect Phobia: A Step-by-Step Guide

By

Trevor Johnson

Introduction

Did you know that 6.1% of the global population suffers from insect phobia? If you're one of them, don't worry - you're not alone. This step-by-step guide is here to help you conquer your fear and regain control.

By understanding your triggers, challenging negative thoughts, and seeking professional help, you can overcome your insect phobia and live a life free from fear.

Let's embark on this journey together and discover a world where insects no longer hold power over you.

Understanding Insect Phobia

To overcome your insect phobia, it's crucial to understand why you feel such intense fear when encountering insects. It's a fear response deeply rooted in our biology and psychology. Our ancestors had to be cautious of insects for survival, as some could be harmful or carry diseases. This fear response, known as entomophobia, can be triggered by a variety of factors, including childhood trauma.

Understanding the fear response is key to overcoming your insect phobia. When you encounter an insect, your brain perceives it as a threat and activates the fight-or-flight response. This leads to a surge of adrenaline, increased heart rate, and heightened senses. It's a natural reaction designed to protect you from danger. However, for some individuals, this fear response becomes exaggerated, causing intense anxiety and panic.

Childhood trauma can also contribute to the development of insect phobia. If you had a negative experience with insects during your formative years, such as being stung or bitten, it can create a lasting impression and trigger fear whenever you encounter insects later in life. It's important to acknowledge and address any past trauma to move forward.

Overcoming childhood trauma is a crucial step in conquering your insect phobia. Professional therapy, such as cognitive-behavioral therapy (CBT), can help you process and reframe your past experiences, allowing you to develop healthier coping mechanisms. Gradual exposure to insects, starting with less threatening ones, can also desensitize your fear response over time.

Identifying Triggers and Symptoms

Understanding the fear response and addressing any childhood trauma are crucial steps in conquering your insect phobia, but now it's time to delve into identifying triggers and symptoms. Identifying triggers is an essential part of managing your phobia. Triggers are the specific situations or stimuli that cause your fear response to kick in. It could be the sight of a particular insect, the sound of buzzing wings, or even the thought of encountering them. By identifying these triggers, you can take steps to avoid or confront them in a controlled manner.

Keep a journal to track your phobia triggers and symptoms. Write down the situations or stimuli that make you feel anxious or fearful. Note down any physical or emotional symptoms you experience when faced with insects. Common symptoms include rapid heartbeat, shortness of breath, sweating, trembling, and feeling a sense of impending doom. By documenting your triggers and symptoms, you can start to recognize patterns and understand what specifically triggers your phobia.

Once you have identified your triggers, it's important to work on managing your symptoms. Deep breathing exercises can help slow down your heart rate and calm your mind when faced with a trigger. Gradual exposure therapy is another effective way to manage your phobia. Start by exposing yourself to your triggers in a controlled environment and gradually increase the intensity as you build up your tolerance. Seeking professional help from a therapist who specializes in phobias can also provide you with guidance and support throughout your journey.

Identifying triggers and managing symptoms are crucial steps in conquering your insect phobia. With time, practice, and support, you can learn to overcome your fear and regain control of your life. Remember, you aren't alone in this journey, and there's help available to guide you every step of the way.

Challenging Negative Thoughts and Beliefs

Now it's time for you to challenge those negative thoughts and beliefs that fuel your insect phobia. Challenging cognitive distortions and reframing negative thoughts are important steps in overcoming your fear. Often, our minds tend to exaggerate the dangers and negative outcomes associated with insects, leading to irrational fears and anxiety. By identifying and challenging these distortions, you can begin to change your perception and response to insects.

One common cognitive distortion is known as catastrophizing, where we automatically assume the worst-case scenario. For example, you may believe that if you encounter a spider, it will surely bite you and cause severe harm. To challenge this thought, ask yourself, 'What evidence do I've to support this belief?' The reality is, most spiders are harmless and avoid human contact. By reminding yourself of this fact, you can begin to reframe your thoughts and reduce the intensity of your fear response.

Another cognitive distortion is known as overgeneralization, where we make broad assumptions based on limited experiences. If you'd a negative encounter with a bee in the past, you may generalize that all bees are dangerous and will sting you. To challenge this belief, remind yourself that not all bees are aggressive and that they play a crucial role in pollination.

Educating yourself about the behavior and characteristics of different insects can help you replace negative thoughts with more accurate and balanced ones.

Seeking Professional Help and Support

Consider reaching out to a mental health professional for guidance and support in overcoming your insect phobia. They can provide you with the professional guidance you need to navigate through the challenges of your phobia. There are various therapy options available that can help you address and manage your fears.

One therapy option that may be recommended is cognitive-behavioral therapy (CBT). CBT focuses on identifying and changing negative thought patterns and behaviors that contribute to your phobia. Through this therapy, you'll learn strategies to challenge and reframe your thoughts about insects, gradually reducing your fear response.

Exposure therapy is another effective treatment for insect phobia. This therapy involves gradually exposing yourself to the object of your fear in a controlled and safe environment. By gradually increasing your exposure to insects, you can desensitize yourself to their presence and reduce your anxiety over time.

Eye movement desensitization and reprocessing (EMDR) therapy is also an option for those struggling with insect phobia. This therapy works by helping you process traumatic experiences associated with insects, allowing you to reframe your thoughts and emotions.

It's important to remember that seeking professional help doesn't mean you're weak or incapable. In fact, it takes strength and courage to acknowledge your fear and take steps towards overcoming it. A mental health professional can provide you with the tools and support you need to face and conquer your insect phobia. Don't hesitate to reach out and seek the help that's available to you.

Learning About Different Insect Species

To better understand and confront your insect phobia, it's helpful to regularly observe and familiarize yourself with various insect species. Learning about different insect species can provide you with valuable knowledge and insights that can help alleviate your fears and anxieties. By understanding their habitats, anatomy, and physiology, you can gain a deeper understanding of these creatures and develop a more rational perspective towards them.

Different insect species have unique habitats that they thrive in. Some insects prefer moist environments, while others prefer dry and arid regions. By learning about the habitats of different insect species, you can better understand where they're commonly found and how to avoid encountering them. Additionally, understanding their habitats can help you appreciate the role they play in the ecosystem and the importance of their existence.

Insect anatomy and physiology can also be fascinating to learn about. By understanding their body structures and functions, you can demystify their behaviors and debunk any misconceptions you may have. For example, learning that most insects don't have the capability to cause harm or transmit diseases can help alleviate fears of being bitten or stung. Additionally, understanding their life cycles and behaviors can help you predict their movements and reduce the likelihood of unexpected encounters.

Regularly educating yourself about different insect species can gradually reduce your phobia by replacing fear with knowledge and understanding. By familiarizing yourself with their habitats, anatomy, and physiology, you can gain a new perspective on these creatures and develop a sense of respect and appreciation for their role in the natural world. Remember, knowledge is power, and the more you learn, the better equipped you'll be to conquer your insect phobia.

Educating Yourself on Insect Behavior

As you continue to familiarize yourself with different insect species, it's essential to consistently observe and study their behavior. Educating yourself on insect behavior can help you overcome your fear and gain a better understanding of these fascinating creatures. Here are some important facts and tips to help you in your journey:

Insect phobia facts:

- Insects play a vital role in maintaining the balance of ecosystems.
- Only a small percentage of insects are harmful to humans.
- Most insects are harmless and are more afraid of you than you're of them.
- Understanding their behavior can help you differentiate between harmless and potentially dangerous species.

Observing insect behavior:

- Take time to watch insects in their natural habitats.
- Observe how they move, communicate, and interact with their surroundings.
- Notice their feeding habits, mating rituals, and defense mechanisms.

- Pay attention to their body language and reactions to different stimuli.

Studying insect behavior:

- Consult reputable sources such as books, documentaries, and websites to learn more about specific insect behaviors.
- Join local insect enthusiast groups or forums to gain insights from experienced individuals.
- Consider taking a course or workshop on entomology to deepen your knowledge.
- Experiment with controlled environments to observe how insects respond to different conditions.

Gradual Exposure Therapy

To overcome your insect phobia, gradually exposing yourself to insects in a controlled environment can be an effective method. Gradual exposure therapy involves exposing yourself to insects in increasing increments, allowing you to gradually build up your tolerance and reduce your fear. This form of therapy has many benefits and can help you overcome the challenges of your phobia.

One of the key benefits of gradual exposure therapy is that it allows you to face your fear in a controlled environment. By starting with less intimidating insects and gradually progressing to more challenging ones, you can build up your confidence and reduce anxiety. This step-by-step approach helps you confront your fear in a manageable way, making it easier to overcome.

Another benefit of gradual exposure therapy is that it helps desensitize your fear response. By repeatedly exposing yourself to insects, your brain begins to rewire itself and recognize that the fear response is unnecessary. Over time, you'll find that your fear diminishes, and you're better able to handle encounters with insects in everyday life.

Of course, overcoming your insect phobia through gradual exposure therapy comes with its own set of challenges. It can be uncomfortable and anxiety-inducing to be in close proximity to insects, especially at the beginning of your therapy. It's important to remember that these challenges are temporary and part of the process. With time and practice, you'll become more comfortable and confident in facing your fear.

Using Relaxation Techniques During Exposure

How can you use relaxation techniques to help you during exposure to insects? When facing your fear of insects, it's crucial to find ways to stay calm and composed. By incorporating relaxation techniques into your exposure therapy, you can effectively manage your anxiety and gradually overcome your phobia. Here are some helpful strategies to try:

- **Visualization techniques**: Visualization involves creating mental images of calm and peaceful scenarios. When you encounter an insect, close your eyes and imagine yourself in a serene and insect-free environment. Picture yourself feeling relaxed and in control. This technique can help shift your focus away from the fear and anxiety, allowing you to feel more at ease.
- **Deep breathing exercises**: Deep breathing is a powerful relaxation tool that can help regulate your heart rate and reduce tension. Take slow, deep breaths in through your nose and exhale slowly through your mouth. As you breathe in, imagine positive energy entering your body, and as you breathe out, visualize the fear and anxiety leaving with each exhale. This technique can help you maintain a sense of calm during exposure to insects.
- **Progressive muscle relaxation**: This technique involves tensing and then releasing each muscle

group in your body, starting from your toes and working your way up to your head. By consciously relaxing your muscles, you can release built-up tension and promote a sense of relaxation.

- **Guided imagery**: Guided imagery involves listening to a recorded script or guide that helps you imagine a specific scenario. Find a guided imagery recording that focuses on overcoming fears or feeling calm in the presence of insects. By following the instructions and visualizations, you can enhance your ability to stay calm during exposure.

Here are some deep breathing exercises that can help you relax and reduce anxiety:

- **4-7-8 Breathing**: Inhale quietly through your nose for a count of 4, hold your breath for a count of 7, and exhale through your mouth for a count of 8. Repeat several times.
- **Box Breathing**: Inhale for a count of 4, hold for 4, exhale for 4, and then rest for 4. Repeat in a square pattern.
- **Diaphragmatic Breathing**: Place one hand on your chest and the other on your abdomen. Inhale deeply through your nose, letting your abdomen rise while keeping your chest relatively still. Exhale through your mouth. This type of breathing engages your diaphragm.
- **Alternate Nostril Breathing**: Close off one nostril with your thumb and inhale deeply

through the other nostril. Then, close off that nostril with your ring finger and release your thumb to exhale through the opposite nostril. Switch and repeat.

- **Belly Breathing**: Lie down and place a small book on your abdomen. Breathe in so that the book rises as you inhale and falls as you exhale.
- **Equal Breathing**: Inhale and exhale for an equal count, such as 4 seconds each. This can help regulate your breath and calm your nervous system.
- **Sama Vritti (Equal Breathing)**: Inhale for a count of 4, then exhale for a count of 4, making your inhales and exhales of equal length.
- **Pursed-Lip Breathing**: Inhale through your nose for two counts and exhale through pursed lips for four counts. This can help calm and lengthen your breath.
- **Guided Breathing**: Listen to guided breathing exercises or meditations, which can walk you through various techniques to help you relax.
- **Breath Counting**: Inhale and count "1," exhale and count "2," inhale and count "3," and so on. Continue until you reach a count of 10, then start over. If your mind wanders, start over from 1.

Remember to practice these deep breathing exercises regularly to experience the most benefit and stress reduction. You can do them anywhere, whether you're sitting at your desk, lying in bed, or taking a short break during the day.

Progressive Muscle Relaxation (PMR) is a technique that involves tensing and then relaxing different muscle groups in the body to help reduce muscle tension and promote relaxation. Here's a step-by-step guide:

- **Find a Quiet Space**: Sit or lie down in a quiet and comfortable place, free from distractions.
- **Start with Your Breath**: Close your eyes and take a few deep breaths to relax.
- **Tense and Relax**: Begin at your feet and work your way up through your body, systematically tensing and relaxing each muscle group. Here's a sample sequence:
    1. Start with your toes. Curl them tightly for a few seconds, then release and relax. Focus on the sensation of relaxation.
    2. Move to your calves. Flex your calf muscles by pointing your toes upward, and then release. Feel the tension leaving your muscles.
    3. Progress to your thighs. Squeeze your thigh muscles for a few seconds, then let go and feel the relaxation.
    4. Continue to your buttocks, then your abdomen, tightening and relaxing each muscle group in turn.
    5. Work your way through your upper body, including your hands, arms, shoulders, neck, and face.
- **Pay Attention to Sensations**: As you release each muscle group, pay attention to the feeling of

relaxation and the contrast between tension and relaxation.

- **Breathe**: Focus on your breath throughout the exercise. Take slow, deep breaths in through your nose and exhale slowly through your mouth. As you exhale, imagine the tension leaving your body.
- **Progressive Sequence**: You can use a sequence that works best for you, or customize it to focus on areas where you carry the most tension.
- **Whole-Body Relaxation**: After you've tensed and relaxed each muscle group, do a final body scan to ensure that your entire body feels relaxed.
- **Stay Relaxed**: Spend a few moments enjoying the relaxed sensation in your body.
- **Practice Regularly**: It's best to practice PMR regularly to benefit from it over time. Some people do it daily as part of a relaxation routine.

Progressive Muscle Relaxation can be a valuable tool for reducing stress and promoting relaxation. By systematically tensing and releasing muscle groups, you become more aware of the physical sensations associated with tension and relaxation, which can help you manage stress and anxiety effectively.

Developing Coping Mechanisms

Incorporate various coping mechanisms to effectively manage your anxiety and gradually overcome your insect phobia. Building resilience and facing your fears head-on are essential steps towards conquering your phobia. Developing coping mechanisms can provide you with the tools to navigate through challenging situations and reduce the intensity of your anxiety.

One effective coping mechanism is cognitive restructuring, which involves changing your negative thought patterns about insects. Challenge your irrational beliefs and replace them with more rational and realistic ones. Remind yourself that most insects are harmless and play important roles in the ecosystem.

Another coping mechanism is exposure therapy, where you gradually expose yourself to insects in a controlled and safe environment. Start with pictures or videos, then progress to observing insects from a distance. As your comfort level increases, you can move on to closer interactions. This gradual exposure allows you to confront your fears in a controlled manner, building resilience and reducing anxiety over time.

Deep breathing exercises and relaxation techniques can also be helpful in managing anxiety. Practice deep breathing to calm your body and mind when you encounter insects. Focus on your breath and try to relax your muscles. This can help you stay grounded and reduce the physical and emotional symptoms of anxiety.

Seeking support from friends, family, or a therapist is crucial in developing coping mechanisms and overcoming your phobia. They can provide understanding, encouragement, and guidance throughout your journey. Remember, you aren't alone, and there are people who are willing to support and help you through this process.

Incorporating coping mechanisms and facing your fears may be challenging, but with perseverance and a willingness to confront your anxiety, you can gradually overcome your insect phobia. By building resilience and utilizing these coping strategies, you can take control of your fears and live a life free from the limitations of phobia.

Building a Support Network

As you continue to develop coping mechanisms, it's important to build a support network that can provide understanding and encouragement throughout your journey of conquering your insect phobia. Building trust and seeking guidance from others who've experienced similar fears can be incredibly beneficial.

Here are some steps to help you build a strong support network:

- **Join a support group**: Look for local or online support groups specifically focused on phobias or anxiety disorders. These groups provide a safe space to share your experiences, learn from others, and receive encouragement from individuals who can relate to your struggles.
- **Connect with loved ones**: Reach out to your friends and family members and let them know about your insect phobia. Opening up about your fears can help them understand what you're going through and allow them to provide the support you need. Their encouragement and presence can make a significant difference in your journey towards overcoming your fear.
- **Seek professional help**: Consider consulting a therapist or counselor specializing in phobias. They can provide guidance and strategies tailored to your specific needs. Therapy sessions can help you explore the root causes of your fear and develop effective coping mechanisms.

- **Engage in exposure therapy**: Exposure therapy is a common treatment for phobias. It involves gradually exposing yourself to the feared object or situation in a controlled and supportive environment. Working with a therapist, you can gradually face your fear of insects and learn to manage your anxiety.

Creating a Safe and Controlled Environment

To create a safe and controlled environment for overcoming your insect phobia, establish a designated space where you can gradually expose yourself to insects under controlled conditions.

Creating a calming atmosphere is crucial in helping you feel more at ease during the exposure exercises.

Start by selecting a room or area in your home where you feel comfortable and safe. Remove any clutter or objects that may trigger anxiety or fear. Make sure the space is well-lit, as darkness can intensify your phobia. Consider adding elements that promote relaxation, such as soft lighting, soothing music, or calming scents like lavender.

Once you have set up the space, it's time to implement exposure exercises. Begin with small steps that gradually expose you to insects. For example, you can start by looking at pictures of insects or watching videos of them from a distance. As you become more comfortable, move on to observing live insects in a controlled environment, such as in a glass container or terrarium.

As you progress, you can introduce more direct interactions with insects. Start by touching objects that have been in contact with insects, such as leaves or twigs. Gradually work your way up to touching insects themselves, using tools like tweezers or gloves if needed. Remember to always prioritize your safety and comfort throughout the process.

By creating a safe and controlled environment and gradually exposing yourself to insects, you can overcome your phobia in a systematic and manageable way. With time and practice, your fear will diminish, and you'll gain confidence in dealing with insects.

Stay patient, be kind to yourself, and celebrate every small achievement along the way. You've got this!

Using Visualization and Positive Affirmations

Once you have established a safe and controlled environment, you can begin using visualization and positive affirmations to further overcome your insect phobia. These techniques help reframe your mindset and build confidence in dealing with your fear. Here are some effective strategies to incorporate into your journey:

- **Visualization techniques:** Visualizing positive scenarios involving insects can help desensitize you to your fear. Close your eyes and imagine yourself calmly observing insects, feeling relaxed and in control. Picture yourself handling insects with ease and confidence. Repeat this exercise regularly to reinforce positive associations.
- **Affirmations and mantras:** Affirmations are powerful statements that can reprogram your subconscious mind. Create affirmations specifically tailored to your phobia, such as 'I am calm and in control around insects' or 'I am becoming more comfortable with insects every day.' Repeat these affirmations daily, both in the presence of insects and during relaxation exercises, to build a sense of empowerment.
- **Breathing exercises:** Deep, slow breathing can help alleviate anxiety and promote relaxation. When faced with an insect or thoughts of insects, take slow, deep breaths in through your nose and

exhale slowly through your mouth. Focus on your breath to divert your attention from your fear and regain a sense of control.

- **Progressive muscle relaxation:** This technique involves tensing and then relaxing each muscle group in your body. Start at your toes, working your way up to your head. As you tense each muscle group, hold it for a few seconds, then release the tension while focusing on the sensation of relaxation. This exercise helps reduce overall tension and promotes a sense of calmness.

Here are some affirmations to consider:

- "I am safe and protected from insects."
- "I am in control of my fear, and I can overcome it."
- "I choose to feel calm and relaxed around insects."
- "Insects play an essential role in nature, and I respect their place in the ecosystem."
- "I release all negative thoughts and fears about insects."
- "I am strong, and I can face my fear of insects with courage."
- "I am learning to coexist peacefully with insects."
- "I trust myself to handle encounters with insects calmly and rationally."
- "I focus on the beauty and diversity of the natural world."

- "I am free from my fear of insects, and I embrace a life without phobia."

You can choose the affirmations that resonate with you the most and repeat them regularly as part of your self-help and exposure therapy for insect phobia. Over time, these positive statements can help shift your mindset and reduce fear and anxiety.

Practicing Mindfulness and Meditation

To continue building upon the techniques discussed in the previous subtopic, incorporate mindfulness and meditation into your journey of conquering your insect phobia. These practices can help you develop a sense of calm and control when faced with your fears.

Mindful breathing is a simple yet powerful technique that can help you ground yourself in the present moment. When you feel anxious or overwhelmed by the presence of insects, take a moment to focus on your breath. Close your eyes if it helps, and take slow, deep breaths, paying attention to the sensation of the breath entering and leaving your body. This practice can help alleviate anxiety and bring you back to a state of calm.

Guided imagery is another effective tool that can be used to overcome your phobia. Close your eyes and imagine yourself in a peaceful and serene environment, such as a lush garden or a tranquil beach. Visualize yourself feeling safe and relaxed in this setting, surrounded by beautiful scenery. As you immerse yourself in this mental imagery, allow yourself to feel the warmth of the sun, the gentle breeze on your skin, and the soothing sounds of nature. This technique can help shift your focus away from your fears and create a sense of peace and tranquility.

Incorporating mindfulness and meditation into your daily routine can help you develop a greater sense of self-awareness and control over your phobia. By practicing mindful breathing and guided imagery, you can cultivate a state of relaxation and ease when faced with insects. Remember, conquering your insect phobia is a journey, and these techniques are tools that can support you along the way. Be patient with yourself and continue to practice these techniques regularly. With time and dedication, you can overcome your fear and live a life free from the constraints of your phobia.

Here's a script to guide you through a relaxation and exposure exercise to help reduce your fear of insects:

Find a quiet and comfortable space where you won't be interrupted. Sit or lie down in a relaxed position. Take a few deep breaths to center yourself.

Progressive Muscle Relaxation:

- Begin by focusing on your breath. Inhale deeply through your nose, and exhale slowly through your mouth. Take a few breaths to calm your body and mind.
- Start at your toes. Tense the muscles in your toes for a few seconds, and then release. Feel the tension melting away as you let go.
- Move up to your feet. Tense the muscles in your feet, and then release. Feel the relaxation spreading through your feet.

- Continue this process, moving up through your body. Tense each muscle group for a few seconds and then release. Work your way through your calves, thighs, abdomen, chest, arms, and up to your neck and head. Allow each area to fully relax before moving on.

Visualizing Exposure:

- Now that you're deeply relaxed, bring to mind a mental image of an insect that you fear. Start with something less intimidating, perhaps a harmless ladybug or butterfly. Picture it in as much detail as you can.
- As you visualize the insect, remind yourself of its harmless nature and the role it plays in the ecosystem. Embrace the idea that it poses no real threat to you.
- Breathe deeply and stay relaxed. Imagine the insect getting closer to you while you remain calm and at ease.
- Gradually, let the insect land on your hand or arm in your visualization. Feel the sensation of it walking gently across your skin without fear.
- If you start to feel anxious or uncomfortable, return to your deep breathing and relaxation exercises.

Positive Affirmations: As you continue the visualization, repeat positive affirmations to reinforce your new mindset:

- "I am safe, and this insect poses no threat to me."
- "I feel calm and relaxed around insects."
- "I respect the role of insects in nature."
- "I am in control of my fears, and I can face them with courage."

When you feel comfortable with this visualization, gradually move on to visualizing encounters with other insects, including those you fear most. Continue to practice this exposure and relaxation technique regularly, and you'll find that your fear of insects diminishes over time.

Remember that overcoming a phobia may take time and persistence. If your phobia is severe, consider seeking support from a mental health professional specializing in exposure therapy or phobia treatment.

Setting Achievable Goals

Continue building upon the techniques discussed in the previous subtopic by setting achievable goals to conquer your insect phobia. Setting goals can provide a sense of direction and purpose, as well as help you track your progress along the way.

By breaking down the process of overcoming your fear of insects into smaller, manageable steps, you can gradually work towards achieving milestones and eventually conquer your phobia. Here are some tips to help you set achievable goals:

- **Start with small, realistic goals:** Begin by setting goals that are within your comfort zone. For example, you can start by looking at pictures of insects or watching videos to desensitize yourself to their presence.
- **Gradually increase the difficulty:** As you become more comfortable with smaller goals, challenge yourself by gradually exposing yourself to more realistic situations. This could involve visiting a butterfly exhibit or observing insects from a distance.
- **Celebrate your achievements:** Recognize and celebrate the milestones you achieve along the way. Each time you successfully confront a fear or complete a goal, reward yourself with something that brings you joy or a sense of accomplishment.

- **Seek support and guidance:** Overcoming obstacles is easier when you have support from others. Consider joining a support group or seeking guidance from a therapist who specializes in phobias. They can provide valuable insights and strategies to help you conquer your insect phobia.

Celebrating Your Progress and Success

As you make progress in conquering your insect phobia, it's important to celebrate your achievements and success. Celebrating milestones along the way can help boost your confidence and motivate you to continue overcoming your fears. Each step you take towards conquering your phobia is a significant accomplishment, no matter how small it may seem.

Take the time to acknowledge and celebrate your progress. Whether it's treating yourself to a small reward, sharing your achievements with a trusted friend or family member, or simply reflecting on how far you've come, these celebrations can reinforce positive feelings and encourage you to keep pushing forward.

Remember that overcoming a phobia is a journey, and it's important to recognize and appreciate the effort and courage it takes to face your fears. By celebrating your progress, you can build a positive mindset and reinforce the belief that you have the ability to conquer your insect phobia.

It can be helpful to set specific milestones or goals along the way, such as being able to spend time in a room with a picture of an insect without feeling anxious, or being able to touch a harmless insect with minimal fear. When you reach these milestones, take the time to celebrate and acknowledge your achievement. This can provide a sense of accomplishment and motivation to continue working towards your ultimate goal of overcoming your insect phobia.

Frequently Asked Questions

Can Insect Phobia Be Completely Cured?

Insect phobia can be completely cured with the right treatments and techniques.

Overcoming fear of insects is a process that requires patience and persistence. By gradually exposing yourself to the source of your fear and learning coping mechanisms, you can gradually reduce your anxiety and eventually conquer your phobia.

It's important to seek professional help or join support groups to guide you through this journey.

How Long Does It Typically Take to Overcome Insect Phobia?

Wondering how long it takes to conquer insect phobia? Well, the time frame can vary depending on the individual. But with the right therapy techniques and dedication, you can make progress sooner than you might think.

Therapy sessions, exposure exercises, and relaxation techniques are commonly used to help overcome this fear. Remember, everyone's journey is unique, so be patient with yourself and celebrate each small step forward.

You've got this!

Are There Any Medications That Can Help With Insect Phobia?

There are alternative medication options and natural remedies that can help with insect phobia. These options can provide relief and support in managing your fear of insects.

Some people find that therapy techniques, such as exposure therapy or cognitive-behavioral therapy, can be effective in reducing phobia symptoms.

Additionally, natural remedies like relaxation techniques, deep breathing exercises, and mindfulness practices can help you cope with anxiety when encountering insects.

It's important to consult with a healthcare professional to determine the best approach for you.

Can Insect Phobia Develop Later in Life?

Late onset phobia, also known as developing a fear of insects later in life, can indeed happen. The causes of late onset phobia can vary from traumatic experiences to a heightened sensitivity to certain stimuli.

It's important to remember that everyone's experiences and fears are unique, and there's no shame in developing a phobia later in life.

Understanding the causes can help you navigate your fear and find strategies to overcome it.

What Are Some Common Misconceptions About Insect Phobia?

So, you want to know about some common misconceptions regarding insect phobia, huh? Well, let's set the record straight.

One big misunderstanding is that people with insect phobia are just being dramatic or overreacting. But trust me, it's not that simple.

Another stereotype is that all insects are creepy and dangerous. But in reality, most bugs are harmless little creatures just trying to live their bug lives. Don't believe the hype, my friend.

Conclusion

Congratulations on taking the courageous steps towards conquering your insect phobia!

By understanding your triggers and challenging negative thoughts, you have embarked on a transformative journey of self-discovery.

Seeking professional help and learning about different insect species have empowered you to face your fears head-on.

Through visualization, mindfulness, and setting achievable goals, you have built resilience and found inner peace.

Remember to celebrate every milestone, for each step forward brings you closer to a life free from the constraints of your phobia.

Keep soaring, brave soul!